DATES MEDICINES

MEDICINES

SHUAIBU ABDULLAHI SAIDU

Copyright © 2022 SHUAIBU ABDULLAHI SAIDU

All rights reserved.

ISBN: **9798361925131**

CONTENTS

001. INTRODUCTION

002. Names & Quran names reference

003. Prophet Abort

004. Scientific benefit

005. Science Hadiths

006. Watermelon & Dates

007. Nutritional value of dates

008. Conclusion

009. about Author

INTRODUCTION

In Sahih Hadith, it is narrated that Prophet Muhammad Sallallaho Alaihe Wasalam said "Whoever ate seven dates in the morning from the area of Aaliyah will not be harmed by poison or magic for the rest of that day". He also said "People of a house where there are no dates are hungry". Prophet Muhammad Sallallaho Alaihe Wasalam ate dried dates with butter, with bread & alone. Tamar is hot in the second degree & either wet or dry in the second degree.

Dried dates strengthen the liver, relax the bowels, increase semen production, especially when taken with pine & relieve soar throat. As for those who are not used to eating dried dates, such as the residents of cold areas, dried dates cause them clogs, harm the teeth & cause headaches, unless they are eaten with almonds & poppy. Dried dates are among the most nutritious fruits; their essence is hot & wet. Also when someone eats dates in the beginning of the day, they help kill worms.

Dried dates are hot & they have the strength of an antidote against worms, killing / decreasing their count, especially when dried dates are taken frequently on an empty stomach. Dried dates are a fruit, type of food, a cure, a drink & a sweet.

Names

1. Latin name is Phoenix dactylifera Linn.

2. Urdu and Hindi name is khajur.

3. English name is dates.

4. Hausa called Dabino

DATES IN ISLAM

Quranic names

1. It is called with various names is Quran.

2. It is called as Nakhl or Nakhil (plural) or Nakhlat (singular) 20 times in Quran.

3. It is called Leenat in chapter Hasr, verse no. 5.

4. It is mentioned asNaqir in chapter Nisa, verse no. 53 and 124.

5. Qitmir in chapter Fatir, verse no. 13.

6. Rutab. In Hadis it is mentioned under 8 names The names mentioned in Hadis are different stages & different varieties of dates Among 8 names, 5 are stages of khajur (dates) & 3 are types of dates. The names in Hadis are

1. Balah -it is a first stage of dates, the dates are unripe (raw) & are not eatable.

2. Bushra– it is the 2nd stage, dates are unripe fresh dates of yellow or red colour & are eatable.

3. Basr– it is the 3rd stage of dates, now the Bushra start getting ripen. They are eatable.

4. Rutab – freshly ripen dates, mainly ripen on its tree. This is what we eat mostly, it is of brownish colour & soft & wet.

5. Tamaar– it the 5th stage of dates, now Rutab gets dried up (mainly on tree).

DATES IN ISLAM

Now the 3 names mentioned in Hadis are, types of dates

1. Barni.
2. Ajwah.
3. Sukhara. Other names in Hadees Bunches of dates are called as Dawaal (دوال) in Hadees. Dates sharbat is called as Nabiz in Hadees. GABA of dates is called as Jimaar (جمار) in Hadees.

Low quality dates are called as Hashaf (حشف) in Hadees. Tamar is mentioned in Hadees as general word for dates. It is important to know about the stages & names mentioned in Hadees.

Quranic references of it

There are 20 references of it in Quran, by the names of **Nakhl** or **Nakhil** (plural) & **Nakhlat** (singular). They are 8 times mentioned alone, and 12 times mentioned with other fruits like pomegranate, grapes, and olives.

1. Chapter **Baqara** verse no. **266**. (Nakhil)

2. Chapter **An'am** verse no. **99**. (Nakhl)

3. Chapter **An'am** verse no. **141**. (Nakhl)

4. Chapter **Ra'ad** verse no. **4**. (Nakhil)

5. Chapter **Nahl** verse no. **11**. (Nakhil)

6. Chapter **Nahl** verse no. **67**. (Nakhil)

7. Chapter **Bani-Israel** verse no. **91**. (Nakhil)

8. Chapter **Khaf** verse no. **32**. (Nakhl)

9. Chapter **Mariam** verse no. **23**. (Nakhlat)

10. Chapter **Mariam** verse no. **25**. (Nakhlat & Rutab)

11. Chapter **Ta'ah** verse no. **71**. (Nakhl)

12. Chapter **Mu-minoon** verse no. **19**. (Nakhil)

13. Chapter **Shu-araa** verse no. **148**. (Nakhl)

14. Chapter **Yaaseen** verse no. **34**. (Nakhil)

15. Chapter **Qaat** verse no. **10**. (Nakhl)

16. Chapter **Qamar** verse no. **20**. **(Nakhl)**

17. Chapter **Rahmaan** verse no. **11**. **(Nakhl)**

18. Chapter **Rahmaan** verse no. **68**. **(Nakhl)**

19. Chapter **Haqqa** verse no. **7**. **(Nakhl)**

20. Chapter **Abasa** verse no. **29**. **(Nakhl)**

Other references of dates in Quran

1. It is referred as **LEENAT** in chapter **HASHR** verse no. 5.

2. In chapter **NISAA** verse no. 53 & 124 it is called as **NAQIR**. (Naqir means a groove or dent on date seed).

3. In chapter **FATIR** verse no. 13 it is called as **QITMIR**. (Qitmir means a groove or dent on dates seed or thin membrane on date seed)

4. In chapter **AN'NAM** verse no. 95 it is called as **NAVA**. (Nava means date seed)

5. In chapter **YASEEN** verse no. 39 it is called **AL-ARJUN**. (Al-Arjun means the lower base of dates which becomes dry & get sickled shaped & it compared with new moon in verse no. 39 of chapter **YASEEN.**

6. In chapter **LAHAB** & **QAMAR** it is called as **HABL** & **DUSUR** (Both means Palm Fibers)

It is important to know about the **stages of date's maturation.**

Because by it only you will understand the uses of it, and why it is called by different names in Quran and Hadis.

DATES IN ISLAM

Stages of dates (According to Growth)

It takes 6 months to get matured and undergo 5 stages. (Means it under go 5 stages on tree or when stored, (before use).
1. **1st stage** of dates is called as **Al-Hababook or Al-saddi.** In this stage the dates are like small balls and are of bitter taste (on tree and are not used).
2. **2nd stage** is called as **Al -Balh.** In this stage the dates are grown little bigger, and are of green colour and pungent it taste. (On tree, and are not used)
3. **3rd stage** is called as **AL -Busr or Al- Khalla**, in this stage the dates get yellowish or reddish colour and turn sweet in taste.

(On tree and can be used but are not used routinely)
4. **4th stage** is called as **Al -Rutab,** now the dates becomes soft, sweet, and get brownish in colour, this stage is ripen stage, and are good to use and was liked by Prophet ﷺ, also it is mentioned in Quran.
5. **5th stage** is called as **Ajwah**. Now the dates get softer, sticky and turn bark brownish. (Also please note Ajwah is also a type of dates and stage of dates.)
6 .**6th stage** is called as **Tamar**, now the dates get dried.

DATES IN ISLAM

Prophet صلى الله عليه وسلم's guidance about dates

Arabic words written in below references are the words mentioned in respected Hadees. You can confirm the references of Hadees at sunna.com & Al-Maktab al-Shamilah(المكتبة الشاملة) also.

Neutralizing hot potency with cold potency: – (Rutab & Bathikh) (Fresh ripen dates & Watermelon): –

1. Hazrat Sahl Bin Saad رضي الله عنه says, that Nabi صلى الله عليه وسلم use to eat Rutab (الرطب) (fresh ripen dates) with Bathikh (البطيخ) (watermelon). : Reference Ibn Ma-jah: 3451; Book No. 29; In English volume no. 4 Book 29, Hadees no 3326.

Also mentioned by Hazrat A'isha رضي الله عنها : Reference Tirmizi: 1843: Book No. 25, Hadees No. 59; In English volume no.3 Book 23, Hadees no 1843.

2. Narrated Hazrat A'isha رضي الله عنها that Nabi صلى الله عليه وسلم said the heat of the one is broken by the coolness of the other, and the coolness of the one by the heat of the other. : Reference Abu Dawud: 3836 Book no. 28; In English Book no. 27; Hadees no. 3827. (This is regarding the above Hadees about eating Rutab dates with watermelon)

DATES IN ISLAM

Tamar & Zubd (dried ripen dates & Butter)

3. Narrated by 2 sons of Busar that Nabi صلى الله عليه وسلم visited Hazrat Busar's home, they presented Tamar (تمر) (dried ripen dates) & Zubd (زبد) (butter) in honor of Nabi صلى الله عليه وسلم because both were liked (together) by Nabi صلى الله عليه وسلم. : Reference Ibn Ma-jah: 3459; Book No. 29; In English volume no. 4 Book 29, Hadees no 3334.
Qissa'a & Rutab (Fresh ripen dates & cucumber): –
4. Hazrat Abdullah Bin Jaffar رضي الله عنه says that Rasool Allah صلى الله عليه وسلم use to eat Qissa'a (القثاء) (cucumber) with Rutab (dates) (الرطب) (fresh ripen dates). : Reference Tirmizi: 1844; Book No. 25; In English volume no. 3 Book 23, Hadees no 1844.
5. Hazrat A'isha رضي الله عنها ate Qissa'a (القثاء) (cucumber) & Rutab (الرطب) (dates) (fresh ripen dates) together to gain weight & she successfully gained weight.

: Reference Ibn Ma-jah: 3449; Book No. 29; In English volume no. 4 Book 29, Hadees no 3324.
Use of Two types of dates together: –
6. Narrated by Jabir Bin Abdullah رضي الله عنه that Nabi صلى الله عليه وسلم prohibited making Nabiz from Basr (البسر) (unripen dates) & Tamar dates together. : Reference Tirmizi: 1876; Book No. 26; In English volume no. 3 Book 24, Hadees no 1876. (Nabiz is prepared by soaking dates in water & drinking that

water, means we should not dip two different types of dates in water & nor drink that sharbat, Nabiz).
7. Hazrat A'isha عنها الله رضي narrated that Rasool Allah وسلم عليہ اللہ صلى said, eat Balah (البلح) (fresh unripen dates) with Tamar (تمر) (dried ripen dates) together (or) old dates with new one & Rasool Allah وسلم عليہ اللہ صلى said, that seeing this shaitaan (الشيطان) gets irritated & the shaitaan (الشيطان) says that human became healthy by eating Balah (البلح) with Tamar (تمر). : Reference Ibn Ma-jah: 3455; Book no. 29; In English volume no. 4 Book 29, Hadees no 3330.
8. Narrated by Jabir Bin Abdullah عنہ الله رضي said that Basr (البسر) (semi ripen) dates with Rutab (الرطب) (fresh ripen dates) are Khamr (intoxicant).

: Reference An-Nasa'I: 5544; Book no. 51; In English Volume 6; Book no. 51; Hadees no. 5546. (Both should not be used together).

(Basr dates (semi ripen) are which start to get ripe, & are yellow or reddish coloured & Rutab dates are which get freshly ripen, (routinely eaten) soft, dark brownish coloured).

Please note we can eat Balah (البلح) (fresh unripen dates) with Tamar (تمر) (dried ripen dates together but we are not allowed to soak both above types of dates to prepare Nabiz because may turn into Alcoholic preparation & please do not soak two types of dates together.

About Rutab Dates

9. Hazrat Sahal Bin Saad رضي الله عنه says that Nabi وسلم عليه الله صلى use to eat Rutab (الرطب) (fresh ripen dates) with Bathikh (البطيخ) (watermelon). : Reference Ibn Ma-jah: 3451; Book no. 29; In English volume no. 4 Book 29, Hadees no. 3326

10. Hazrat Abdullah Bin Jaffar رضي الله عنه says that Rasool Allah وسلم عليه الله صلى use to eat Qissa'a (القثاء) (cucumber) with Rutab (dates) (الرطب) (fresh ripen dates). : Reference Tirmizi: 1844; Book No. 25; In English volume no.3 Book 23, Hadees no 1844.

11. Hazrat A'isha رضي الله عنها ate Qissa'a (القثاء) (cucumber) & Rutab (الرطب) (dates) (fresh ripen dates) together to gain weight & she successfully gained weight. : Reference Ibn Ma-jah: 3449; Book no. 29;In English volume no. 4 Book 29, Hadees no. 3324.

About Tamar Dates

The word Tamar may be used for a type of date (dried ripen dates) or commonly for routine dates.

12. Narrated Hazrat A'isha رضي الله عنها that Nabi صلى الله عليه وسلم said heat of the one is broken by the coolness of the other, and the coolness of the one by the heat of the other. :

Reference Abu Dawud: 3836 Book no. 28; In English Book no. 27; Hadees no. 3827. (This is regarding the above Hadees about eating Rutab dates with watermelon).

13. Narrated by 2 sons of Busar that Nabi صلى الله عليه وسلم visited Hazrat Busar's home, they presented Tamar (تمر) (dried ripen dates) & Zubd (زبد) (butter) in honor of Nabi صلى الله عليه وسلم because both were liked (together) by Nabi صلى الله عليه وسلم : Reference Ibn Ma-jah: 3459; Book No. 29;In English volume no.4 Book 29, Hadees no 3334.

14. Hazrat Aamir Bin Saad Abu Waqqas رضي الله عنه heard from his father that Nabi صلى الله عليه وسلم said that anyone who eats 7 Tamar (تمر) (dates) daily, which grow between these two lava plains (two Madinah (المدينه) mountains) empty stomach, early morning, than till evening, will not be affected with poisoning (سم) & black magic (سحر) (witch craft) & if eats at evening, will safe from poison (سُمّ) & black magic (سحر) (witch craft) till morning. : Reference Muslim: 2047 A; Book no. 36; In English Book no. 23; Hadees no. 5080.

15. Hazrat Abu Hurairah رضي الله عنه says that Nabi

وسلم عليہ اللہ صلى said by eating Tamar (تمر) (dates), Qalounj (القولنج) will not occur. : Reference Abu Nuaim: 828. Qalounj (القولنج): – it is a condition in which people suffer from inferior complex due to strictures, obstructions, spasm or pain.

16. Hazrat Abdullah Ibn Abbas رضي الله عنه says that Rasool Allah وسلم عليہ اللہ صلى guided that eat Tamar (تمر) (dates) on empty stomach early morning, by this worm of stomach get killed. : Reference Musnad Firdous: 4813.

DATES IN ISLAM

Jaw chapatti (bread) & Tamar dates

17. Hazrat Yusuf Ibn Abdullah Ibn Salam عنه الله رضي says that he saw Nabi وسلم عليه الله صلى eating jaw (barley flour) chapatti (Bread) (خبز) with Tamar (تمر) (dried ripen dates) & said that dates (تمر) are equivalent to gravy with jaw (barley) chapatti (Bread).
 : Reference Abu Dawud: 3830; Book no. 28; In English book no. 27; Hadees no. 3821.
Discipline while eating in company of people: –
18. Hazrat Abdullah Bin Umar عنه الله رضي reported that Nabi وسلم عليه الله صلى said, do not pick more than one dates at the time, nor pick 2 or more to eat, without permission, (when we are eating in company of people).   : Reference Tirmizi: 1814, Book no. 25; In English volume no. 3 Book No. 23, Hadees no 1814.
A position of sitting while eating dates: –
19. Hazrat Anas Bin Malik عنه الله رضي says that he saw Nabi وسلم عليه الله صلى eating Tamar (تمر) (dried ripen dates) in sitting position on heels. : Reference Muslim: 2044 a; Book no. 36; In English Book no. 23; Hadees no 5073.

Hasis (Hais) (a sweet dish)

20. Narrated by Hazrat Anas Bin Malik رضي الله عنه that Nabi صلى الله عليه وسلم married Hazrat Safiya رضي الله عنها & called people for a feast (as dawat e valima) & served people with Hais, (Hasis) on a piece of leather (dastarkhaan). : Reference Bukhari: 5387; Book No. 70; In English volume no. 7 Book no. 65; Hadees no 299.
Hais (Hasis) is a sweet dish (halwa) prepared from Tamar (تمر) dates, milk, jaw (barley), ghee, paneer etc.

DATES IN ISLAM

Importance of having dates in house

21. Hazrat A'isha عنها الله رضي says that Nabi اللہ صلی علیہ وسلم said that a family which has dates (Tamar) will not be hungry. : Reference Muslim: 2046 a; Book no. 36; In English Book no. 23; Hadees no. 5078.
22. Narrated Hazrat A'isha عنها الله رضي that Rasool Allah وسلم علیہ اللہ صلی said the house which do not have dates (تمر) those people are (will be) hungry. :

Reference Tirmizi: 1815, Book no. 25; In English volume no. 3 Book No. 23, Hadees no 1815
23. Narrated by Ubaidullah from his grandmother Salma عنها الله رضي says that Nabi وسلم علیہ اللہ صلی said that the house which does not have dates (تمر) the house is as, there is no food. : Reference Ibn Ma-jah: 3453; Book no. 29; In English volume no. 4 Book 29, Hadees no 3328.

Dates & Dinner

24. Narrated by Anas Bin Malik عنه الله رضي that Nabi وسلم عليه الله صلى said that Always eat dinner & if you have nothing to eat, at least eat few Hashaf (حشف) (low quality dates) (or handful of something to eat) because skipping dinner will make you old & weak. : Reference Tirmizi: 1856; Book No. 25, Hadees No. 73; In English volume no.3 Book 23, Hadees no 1856.

25. Narrated by Jabir Bin Abdullah عنه الله رضي that Nabi وسلم عليه الله صلى said never skip dinner, though you only have few Tamar (dates) (تمر), eat them because skipping dinner will make you old. : Reference Ibn Ma-jah: 3480; Book no. 29; In English volume no. 4 Book 29, Hadees no 3355.

Old dates

26. Narrated by Anas Bin Malik رضي الله عنه that somebody presented some old dates to Nabi صلى الله عليه وسلم & Nabi صلى الله عليه وسلم started opening the dates (تمر) (Tamar) to see (the worm) . : Reference Ibn Ma-jah: 3458; Book no. 29; In English Book 29, Hadees no 3333

Half ripen dates (Basr): –

27. Hazrat Abu A'seeb رضي الله عنه says, that one night Nabi صلى الله عليه وسلم took Hazrat Abu Aaib, Abu Bakr, Umar رضي الله عنه to An Ansari's dates garden & asked the owner of the garden to give Basr (بسر) (half ripen dates), the owner went & brought branches of dates & all ate to their satisfaction. : Reference Musnad Ahmed: 20787.

About Ajwah Dates

28. Hazrat Ra'fe Bin Umar Al Majni عنه الله رضي says, that Rasool Allah وسلم عليه الله صلى said that Ajwah (العجوة) & Saukhara (الصخرة) both are from Jannah (الجنة). : Reference Ibn Ma-jah: 3583; Book no. 31; In English volume no. 4 Book 31, Hadees no 3456.

29. Hazrat A'isha عنها الله رضي says that Rasool Allah وسلم عليه الله صلى guided that The Ajwah dates of 'Aliya' contain healing effects and these are antidote (for poisoning) if eaten early morning   : Reference Muslim : 2048; Book no. 36; In English Book no. 23; Hadees no. 5083.

30. Hazrat Saad عنه الله رضي says that Rasool Allah وسلم عليه الله صلى guided that eat 7 Ajwah (عجوة) (dates) early morning empty stomach, that day, the person will be saved from poisoning (سم) & black Magic (سحر) (witch craft). : Reference Bukhari: 5769; Book No. 76; In English volume no. 7 Book no. 71; Hadees no 664.

31. Hazrat A'isha عنها الله رضي says that Nabi صلى الله عليه وسلم guided to use 7 Ajwah (عجوة) (dates) of Madinah (المدينه) for 7 days; this helps in curing Juzam (الجزام). : Reference Abu Nu-aim: 899.   (Juzam is kodh) (Leprosy).

32. Hazrat Sa'ad Bin Abi Waqqas عنه الله رضي says that he fell ill, he had chest pain, Rasool Allah صلى الله عليه وسلم visited him & kept his respected palm on Hazrat Sa'ad عنه الله رضي chest, Hazrat Sa'ad عنه felt the soothing effect in his whole chest & Rasool Allah وسلم عليه الله صلى prayed for him, & said that Sa'ad is suffering from cardiac problem. And

Rasool Allah وسلم عليه الله صلى advised to take Hazrat Sa'ad عنه الله رضي to Haris Bin Kuladah (a hakim) and said the physician should give 7 Ajwah (عجوة) (dates) of Madinah (المدينه) crushed, & with its seed grinded & put it in your mouth. : Reference Abu Dawud: 3875; Book no. 29; In English Book no. 28; Hadees no 3866.

Cure for Poisoning

33. Narrated by Hazrat Abu Hurairah عنه الله رضي that Nabi وسلم عليه الله صلى said that Ajwah (عجوة) (dates) are from Jannah (الجنة) & in it there is cure (شفاء) for poisoning (سم), And Kamaat (الكماة) (Mushrooms or Truffles) are among Mann (المن) (a reward) & its water is cure (شفاء) for eye (العين) diseases. : Reference Tirmizi: 2208; Book No. 28, In English volume no. 4, Hadees no 2066.

Jimaar (Gaba of dates) & Palm Date tree & Muslims

34. Hazrat Abdullah Bin Umar رضي الله عنه says that we were sitting with Nabi صلى الله عليه وسلم Jimaar (جمار) (Gaba of dates) was sent by someone, than Nabi صلى الله عليه وسلم asked "Among all trees, which tree is like Muslim & Allah Ta'lah has given Barkat in it?" (As barkat Muslims have) than Nabi صلى الله عليه وسلم answered (himself) that it is Nakhl (النخلة) (palm date tree). : Reference Bukhari: 5444; Book no. 70; In English volume no. 7 Book no. 65; Hadees no 355. (Jimaar is GABA of dates; it is obtained from gum of dates trees).

Guidance about Dates After illness & during illness

35. Hazrat Umme Munzir رضي الله عنها says that, Rasool Allah صلى الله عليه وسلم & Hazrat Ali رضي الله عنه both came home, she had Dawaal (دوال) (bunches of dates), she served Dawaal (دوال) to both, both started to eat the dates, but when Hazrat Ali رضي الله عنه had eaten 7 dates (approximately) he was stopped by Rasool Allah صلى الله عليه وسلم from eating more, & said to Hazrat Ali رضي الله عنه that you were ill last days & now you are weak, so do not eat more, Hearing to his Hazrat Umme Munzir رضي الله عنها prepared Sareed (ثرد) (thin gravy) of meat, beet root & chapatti (خبز) from Jaw (الشعير) (barely flour) & served to both, on this Rasool Allah صلى الله عليه وسلم said to Hazrat Ali

رضي الله عنه eat this dish, this is beneficial for you. :
Reference Tirmizi: 2170; Book No. 28; In English
volume no. 4, Book 2, Hadees no 2036.
36. Hazrat Suhaib رضي الله عنه reports that his right eye
was paining & he was eating Tamar (تمر) (dates),
looking to this; Rasool Allah صلى الله عليه وسلم said that,
you are eating Tamar (تمر) (dates) in spite of eye pain,

On this Hazrat Suhaib
رضي الله عنه said that I am eating from left side & my
right eye is paining. : Reference Baihaqi : 20047.

About Barni dates
37. Hazrat Anas Bin Malik رضي الله عنه says that Nabi
صلى الله عليه وسلم said that among the Tamar (تمر)
(dates) you have, Barni (البرني) (it is a type of dates)
are the best, there is cure for diseases in it & have no
harmful effects. : Reference Mustadrak Al Hakim:
7450.

About breaking fast
38. Salman Bin 'Amr رضي الله عنه narrated Nabi صلى
الله عليه وسلم guided us to break the fast with Tamar (تمر)
(dates) & if dates are not present than break the fast
with water because water is pure (paak). :
Reference Ibn Ma-jah: 1769; Book no. 7; In English
volume no. 1; Book no. 7; Hadees no. 1699.
39. Hazrat Anas Bin Malik رضي الله عنه says that
Rasool Allah صلى الله عليه وسلم use to break the fast
before Magrib Salah with Rutab (الرطب) (fresh ripen
dates) or old dates which ever would be present, if
dates would not be present, than broke the fast with
water. : Reference Abu Dawud: 2356; Book no.14; In
English Book no. 13; Hadees no. 2349.

About Tahneek

40. Hazrat Asma Bint Abu Bakr عنها الله رضي gave birth to a son (in Yuba), this birth was the first birth in Muslim society, Means, that time the Yahudis of Madinah had challenged the Muslims, that due to their Black magic none Muslim lady will give birth to any child, On the birth of her son (Abdullah Bin Zubair عنه الله رضي) all Muslims gathered & sang slogans of Takbir loudly. Hazrat Asma Bint Abu Bakr عنها الله رضي took the infant to Rasool Allah وسلم عليه الله صلى, Rasool Allah وسلم عليه الله صلى took the infant in his respected laps & called for Tamar (تمر) (dates) & chewed the dates & spat it into the infant's mouth & rubbed it on the upper palate of the infant & prayed for Barkat. : Reference Bukhari: 5469; Book no. 71; In English volume no. 7, Book no. 66; Hadees no 378. The above act of dates to be spatted & rubbed on infant's upper palate is called as TAHNEEK.
41. Hazrat Abu Moosa Ashari عنه الله رضي says that Tahneek was done by Nabi وسلم عليه الله صلى to his infant, & also Rasool Allah وسلم عليه الله صلى named his infant as Ibrahim (ابراهيم). : Reference Bukhari: 5467; Book no. 71; In English volume no. 7, Book no. 66; Hadees no 376.

Tahneek

It is to take a date or something sweet in our mouth & chew it a little, than put the date or the sweet thing into new born's mouth & rub the date at upper palate of new born's mouth for a while. Nabi وسلم عليه الله صلى use to do it, this is a sunnat, which we should do it. Now days, new born suffer from juvilian diabetes &

lack of glucose, which causes brain damage of new born, this sunnat, we can solve many problems of new born.

Dried Grapes & Tamar dates together prohibited

42. Hazrat Jabir Bin Abdullah عنه الله رضي reported that Nabi وسلم عليه الله صلى prohibited the mixing of dried grapes (Zabib) and dates (Tamar), and dry dates (Tamar) and (Basr) fresh dates. : Reference Muslim: 1986 A; Book no. 36; In English Book no. 23; Hadees no. 4896.

43. Nabi وسلم عليه الله صلى guided, do not combine fresh dates and unripe dates, or raisins and dates; rather make Nabiz with each one of them on its own." (Separately). : Reference Ibn Ma-jah: 3523; Book no. 30; In English volume no. 4 Book 30, Hadees no 3397.

About Nabiz

According to many references & scholars, Nabi صلى وسلم عليه الله liked Nabiz very much. Nabiz is, dates or raisins soaked overnight in water & this water (sharbat) should be drunk & this sharbat is called as Nabiz. But do not soak two types of dates together nor dates with raisins.

44. Hazrat Sahl Bin Sa'ad عنه الله رضي narrates that Abu Usaid As-Sa'di عنه الله رضي invited Rasool Allah وسلم عليه الله صلى at his Valima feast (wedding party) & after meal nabiz was given to Nabi وسلم عليه الله صلى to drink. : Reference Bukhari: 5176; Book no. 67; In English volume no. 7; Book no.62; Hadees no.105.

45. Narrated by Jabir Bin Abdullah عنه الله رضي that Nabi وسلم عليه الله صلى prohibited making nabiz from Basr (البسر) (unripen dates) & Tamar dates together. :

Reference Tirmizi: 1876; Book No. 26; In English volume no. 3, Book 24, Hadees no 1876. (Nabiz is prepared by dipping dates in water & drinking the water means we should not dip two different types of dates in water).

46. Narrated by Abu Saeed عنه الله رضي that Nabi صلى وسلم عليه الله prohibited mixing of unripen dates & dates together, & mixing of Raisins & dates for making Nabiz & prohibited the jars that Nabiz is made in. : Reference Tirmizi: 1877; Book No. 26, Hadees No. 17; In English volume no. 3 Book 24, Hadees no 1877.

47. Nabi وسلم عليه الله صلى prohibited to prepare Nabiz if the following: earthen pots, Dubba (pumpkin), trunk of palm dates tree, coated pitch, green pot & said I forbid you to use the above, but they do not make anything lawful nor unlawful, but ever intoxicant is unlawful. : Reference Tirmizi: 1867, 1868, 1869; Book No. 26; In English volume no. 3, Book 24, Hadees no 1867, 1868, and 1869. (Means Nabiz gets toxic or alcoholic by the above means).

48. Narrated by A'isha عنها الله رضي that we use to prepare Nabiz for Nabi وسلم عليه الله صلى in a water Skin (water bag) which was tie at the top & it had a small hole in it, Nabiz prepared in morning was drank at evening & which was prepared at evening was drank at morning. : Reference Tirmizi: 1871; Book No. 26; In English volume no.3; Book 24, Hadees no 1871.

A Feast

49. Hazrat Anas عنه الله رضي says that once my mother Umme Sulem عنها الله رضي ask me to give a basket of dates to Rasool Allah وسلم عليه الله صلى, Hazrat Anas عنه الله رضي went to Rasool Allah صلى الله عليه

DATES IN ISLAM

وسلم's home, but he came to know that Rasool Allah وسلم عليہ اللہ صلى has gone to a feast at his ex-slave to whom Nabi وسلم عليہ اللہ صلى had freed in past.

(Actually Nabi وسلم عليہ اللہ صلى had freed this slave; the slave became a good tailor & earned good money for himself. Now he had invited Nabi وسلم عليہ اللہ صلى for a feast along with some companions of Nabi وسلم عليہ اللہ صلى).

When Hazrat Anas عنہ اللہ رضي reach the slave's place, everybody was eating, Hazrat Anas عنہ اللہ رضي was asked to join the feast & he did. They were served with Sareed (ثرد) made from pumpkin (kara'a), dried meat & jaw (barley) chapatti. Hazrat Anas رضي اللہ عنہ knew that pumpkin (kara'a) was favourite to Rasool Allah وسلم عليہ اللہ صلى & he use to collect pieces of pumpkin (kara'a) in front of Rasool Allah صلى اللہ عليہ وسلم. Than after the feast, Hazrat Anas عنہ اللہ رضي & Rasool Allah وسلم عليہ اللہ صلى went to Rasool Allah وسلم عليہ اللہ صلى's home & Hazrat Anas عنہ اللہ رضي gave the basket of dates. (The respected) Rasool Allah وسلم عليہ اللہ صلى was eating the dates & distributing the dates among people, till the dates finished. : Reference Bukhari: 5379 & 5420; Book no. 70; In English volume no. 7 Book no. 65; Hadees no 291 & 331. : Reference Ibn Ma-jah: 3428; Book no. 29; In English volume no. 4; Book 29, Hadees no 3303. (& also from other reference all are mixed & written, please note).

DATES IN ISLAM

QURAN reciting people

50. Hazrat Abu Musa Al-Ash'ari عنه الله رضي says that Rasool Allah وسلم عليه الله صلى said " believer who recites the Qur'an is like an orange whose fragrance is sweet and whose taste is sweet, a believer who does not recite the Qur'an is like a date which has no fragrance but has a sweet taste and the hypocrite (munafiq & faajir) who recites the Qur'an is like (Rehaan) basil whose fragrance is sweet, but whose taste is bitter
and a hypocrite (munafiq & faajir) who does not recite the Qur'an is like the colocynth which has no fragrance and has a bitter taste. : Reference Bukhari: 5427; Book no. 70; In English volume no. 7, Book no. 65; Hadees no 338. (Colocynth is a bitter cucumber & also bitter apple).

For praise Allah
51. Narrated by Anas Bin Malik عنه الله رضي that Nabi وسلم عليه الله صلى said:" Indeed Allah is pleased with the slave who, upon eating his food or drinking his drink, he praises Him for it". : Reference Tirmizi: 1816; Book no. 25; In English volume no. 3 Book No. 23, Hadees no 1816.

Rutab dates for Menstrual Problems
52. Hazrat Abu Hurairah عنه الله رضي says, that Nabi وسلم عليه الله صلى said, that in my knowledge Rutab (الرطب) (fresh ripen dates) are best remedy for excessive menstrual flow & Honey (العسل) is best for patients (المريض). : Reference Abu Nu-aim 459.

A preparation with Hulba (Methi) for sick person

53. Once Hazrat Saad Bin Abi Waqqas رضي الله عنه fell ill in Makkah, Nabi صلى الله عليه وسلم visited him, and asked to call a doctor, Al Haris Bin Kuladah was called, he came and examined Hazrat Saad رضي الله عنه, and said he is not serious, and advised to take dates (khajur), barley (jaw) & boiled Methi water & prepare daliya (soup like gravy) than put honey on it & give to Hazrat Saad رضي الله عنه at early morning, garma-garam (warm). And Hazrat Saad رضي الله عنه got well; Nabi صلى الله عليه وسلم liked the preparation advised by Al Haris Bin Kuladah. : Reference At-tibbe Nabawi Harful Haa volume no. 1; page no. 230.

54. Hazrat Sa'ad Bin Abi Waqqas رضي الله عنه says that he fell ill, he had chest pain, Rasool Allah صلى الله عليه وسلم visited him & kept his respected palm on Hazrat Sa'ad رضي الله عنه chest, Hazrat Sa'ad رضي الله عنه felt the soothing effect in his whole chest & Rasool Allah صلى الله عليه وسلم prayed for him, & said that Sa'ad is suffering from cardiac problem. And Rasool Allah صلى الله عليه وسلم advised to take Hazrat Sa'ad رضي الله عنه to Haris Bin Kuladah (a hakim) And Rasool Allah صلى الله عليه وسلم said the physician should give 7 Ajwah (عجوة) (dates) of Madinah (المدينه) crushed, & with its seed grinded & put it in your mouth. : Reference Abu Dawud: 3875; Book no. 29; In English Book no. 28; Hadees no 3866.

Gaba of dates (Jimaar) (جمار)

It is called Jimaar & Shaham Annakhal in Arabic, & in Hadees it is called as Jimaar (جمار), it is obtained from date tree, it is gum of palm date tree. It is used for the following: -Loose motion, chest pain, TB, throat infection, soar voice, cough & cold, it makes the intestine strong, strengthens the body, makes blood pure, reduces swelling of kidneys, maintains general health, removes weakness, can be applied on wounds, But first the gum should be purified & than used.

Content of dates

Glucose, sugar, vitamin A, vitamin B1, B2, B3, B12, calcium, phosphate, potassium, sulphur, sodium, magnesium, cobalt, zinc, fluorine, copper, manganese, cellulose, fructose, biotin, amino acids, fibers, carbohydrates, water, fats, iron, etc. Fresh dates have pitocin hormone which helps in delivery, it contracts the uterus.

Scientific benefits of dates

1. Helps in constipation.
2. Delivery. (Fresh dates)
3. Have great nutritive values.
4. Nourishes the brain.
5. Improves the peristalsis movement of intestine.
6. It forms RBC, bone marrow, haemoglobin thus good in anaemia & etc.
7. Maintains pH level of blood.
8. Reduces weight, fats and slims the body.
9. Protects against cancer.
10. Increases urine output, libido.
11. Strengthens the bone, teeth, eye sight, and ear nerves.
12. Reduces thyroid activity, so helpful in

hyperthyroidism.
13. Helpful for liver function, dry lips, dry skin, cracked nails etc.
14. Improves function of bladder, stomach and intestines.
15. Best for pregnant.
16. Helps in kidney stones, gall stones, gouts, blood pressure, piles.etc

Science & Hadees regarding Dates

Prophet صلى الله عليه وسلم said, "Whoever takes seven 'Ajwah dates in the morning will not be effected by magic or poison on that day." Nabi صلى الله عليه وسلم has also said, "There is a tree among the trees which is similar to a Muslim (in goodness), and that is the date palm tree." As Muslims we are wise to include these foods in our diet. Allah has blessed us with many good foods and in the Quran (7:160) it says "Eat of the good foods We have provided for you." Prophet صلى الله عليه وسلم used to break the fast by eating some dates before offering Magrib (sunset) prayer, and if ripe dates were not available, he used to substitute them with some dried grapes. When they too were not available, he used to have a few sips of water, according to some reports. Modern science has proved that dates are part of a healthy diet. They contain sugar, fat and proteins, as well as important vitamins. Hence the great importance attached to them by the Prophet صلى الله عليه وسلم.

Dates are also rich in natural fibers. Modern medicine has shown that they are effective in preventing abdominal cancer. They also surpass other fruits in the sheer variety of their constituents. They contain oil, calcium, sulphur, iron, potassium, phosphorous, manganese, copper and magnesium. In other words, one date is the equivalent of a balanced and healthy diet. Arabs usually combine dates with milk and yogurt or bread, butter (A sweet dish called as Hais is sunnat & beloved to Prophet صلى الله عليه وسلم). This combination indeed makes a balanced and nutritious diet for both mind and body. Dates and date palms have been mentioned in the Holy Quran nearly 20 times, thus showing their importance. The Prophet صلى الله عليه وسلم likened a good Muslim to the date palm, saying: "Among trees, there is a tree like a Muslim. Its leaves do not fall."

Maryam (Mary) (a.s), the mother of Jesus was advised to eat dates as her food when she felt labor pains, during her confinement. Dates are definitely the "crown of sweets," and an ideal food which is easy to digest, and within half an hour of taking it, the tired body regains vigor. The reason for this is that a shortage of sugar in the blood is the main factor that makes people feel hungry and not an empty stomach as is often assumed. When the body absorbs the nutritional essence of a few dates, the feeling of hunger becomes appeased. Breaking the fast with

dates helps one avoid over-eating later.
Experiments have also shown that dates contain some stimulants that strengthen the muscles of the uterus in the last months of pregnancy. This helps the dilation of the uterus at the time of delivery on one hand and reduces the bleeding after delivery on the other. Dieticians consider dates as the best food for women in confinement and those who are breast-feeding. This is because dates contain elements that assist in alleviating depression in mothers and enriching the breast-milk with all the elements needed to make the child healthy and resistant to disease. Prophet صلى الله عليه وسلم has emphasized the importance of dates and their effectiveness in the growth of the fetus. He has also recommended they be given to women. Modern dietitians now recommend dates to be given to children suffering from nervous disorders or hyperactivity. The Prophet صلى الله عليه وسلم has also recommended dates as a medicine for heart troubles, according to some reports. Modern science has also proved the effectiveness of date, in preventing diseases of the respiratory system. Cucumber & dates together: –
3. Cucumber & dates: cumber has a cold effect and dates have a hot one. By combining the two it becomes mild. From this Hadees we gather that it is recommended that the effect (hot or cold) of things eaten should be taken into consideration. Cucumber is insipid and tasteless, and dates are sweet which results in the cucumber also tasting sweet. Both are

DATES IN ISLAM

opposite to each other cucumber are rich in water contains.

4. Please match the nutritional facts of both cucumber & dates & see what a combination both is, both makes a perfect nutrition & opposite to each other. This is the miracle of sunnat of Prophet ﷺ eating both together.

Nutritional value of Cucumber. 100 grams of dates has 16 calories only. Water content is cucumber is 96%.

Total Fat 0.1 g	0%
Saturated fat 0 g	0%
Polyunsaturated fat 0 g	
Monounsaturated fat 0 g	
Cholesterol 0 mg	0%
Sodium 2 mg	0%
Potassium 147 mg	4%
Total Carbohydrate 3.6 g	1%
Dietary fiber 0.5 g	2%
Sugar 1.7 g	
Protein 0.6 g	1%

Vitamin A 2%   Vitamin C 4%   Calcium 1%
Iron 1%   Vitamin D 0%   Vitamin B6 10%
Magnesium 3% Nutritional value of dates. 100 grams of dates has 282 calories. Water content is dry dates 10% to 20%.

Total Fat 0.4 g	0%
Saturated fat 0 g	0%

Polyunsaturated fat 0 g
Monounsaturated fat 0 g
Cholesterol 0 mg   0%
Sodium 2 mg   0%
Potassium 656 mg   18%
Total Carbohydrate 75 g   25%
Dietary fiber 8 g   32%
Sugar 63 g
Protein 2.4 g   4%
Vitamin A 0%   Vitamin C %   Calcium 3%
Iron 5%   Vitamin D 0%   Vitamin B6 10%
Magnesium 10%

Watermelon & Dates together

Nutritional value of watermelon. 100 grams of dates has 30 calories only

Water content is dry dates 92%

Total Fat 0.2 g	0%
Saturated fat 0 g	0%
Polyunsaturated fat 0 g	
Monounsaturated fat 0 g	
Cholesterol 0 mg	0%
Sodium 1 mg	0%
Potassium 112 mg	18%
Total Carbohydrate 8 g	25%

Dietary fiber 0.4 g   32%

Sugar 6 g

Protein 0.6 g   4%

Vitamin A 11%   Vitamin C 13%   Calcium 0%

Iron 1%   Vitamin D 0%   Vitamin B6 0%

Magnesium 2%

Nutritional value of dates. 100 grams of dates has 282 calories.

Water content is dry dates 10% to 20%.

Total Fat 0.4 g   0%

Saturated fat 0 g   0%

Polyunsaturated fat 0 g

Monounsaturated fat 0 g

Cholesterol 0 mg   0%

Sodium 2 mg   0%

Potassium 656 mg   18%

Total Carbohydrate 75 g   25%

Dietary fiber 8 g   32%

Sugar 63 g

Protein 2.4 g   4%

Vitamin A 0%   Vitamin C %   Calcium 3%

Iron 5%   Vitamin D 0%   Vitamin B6 10%

Magnesium 10%

5. Match the nutrition of both & judge both are opposite to each other & both in combination make a perfect nutrition. This is miracle of Sunnats of Prophet صلى الله عليه وسلم eating both together.

Conclusion

1. Eat fresh ripen dates & watermelon or Mashmelon together because one cools the other. Eat butter & dried dates together, cucumber & dates, Balah (fresh unripen dates) & Tamar (dried dates).

2. Avoid making Nabiz from two types of dates or dates & raisins, semi ripen dates & ripen dates together are Khamr (intoxicant). 7 Ajwah dates eaten early morning empty stomach prevents black magic, evil eye, cardiac problems, skin disease & Ajwah dates are from Jannah.

3. Dates if eaten on early morning empty stomach are helpful in worms, inferior complex. Keep dates always at home & it has Barkat in it as Muslims have. Do not pick more than 1 dates at a time to eat, do not eat excessively during or after illness, 7 dates at one time are best. They are best nutrition, do Tahneek to new born with dates.

DATES IN ISLAM

ABOURT AUTHOR

The author's name is Shuaibu Abdullahi Sa'idu, he was born in Gombe, Nigeria. He was born on 01/12/1999. He has been living in Gombe for the past twenty-three years in a neighborhood called (sirankiyo). They migrated. Before that, they lived in neighborhoods like this. First, where he was born, the name of the neighborhood (Pantami) they left this neighborhood and moved to another neighborhood called (Hammadu kafi) this is it

www.ingramcontent.com/pod-product-compliance
Lightning Source LLC
Chambersburg PA
CBHW050318220526
45465CB00005B/2037